REVITALIZE YOUR SKIN WITH ORGANIC SOAP:

Homemade Recipes for Healthy and Youthful Skin in 2023

Lily Rose

Table of contents

Chapter 1

Introduction to Soap Making

Organic soap making is the art of creating soap using natural and organic ingredients, without the use of synthetic fragrances, harsh chemicals, or potentially harmful additives. The process involves combining plant-based oils, such as olive, coconut, or palm oil, with an alkaline solution, typically sodium hydroxide (also known as lye). This chemical reaction, known as saponification, produces soap, a cleansing and moisturizing substance that has been used for thousands of years.

The use of organic soap has gained popularity in recent years as more people become aware of the potential risks associated with commercial soaps that contain synthetic chemicals and irritants. Organic soap making allows individuals to create soap that is gentle and nourishing for the skin, while also promoting sustainable and environmentally conscious practices.

Soap making can be done using different methods, including cold process, hot process, and melt and pour. Each method has its own advantages and challenges, and soap makers can choose the one that best suits their preferences and skill level. Homemade soap can also be customized with various essential oils, herbs, botanicals, and natural colorants, to create unique and therapeutic blends that are tailored to individual needs and preferences.

In summary, organic soap making is a rewarding and creative process that allows individuals to make soap that is healthy for the skin and the environment, using natural and sustainable ingredients. With the right knowledge, tools, and techniques, anyone can learn to make their own homemade soap and enjoy the benefits of this ancient and versatile cleansing agent.

Chapter 2

Benefits of Organic Soap

Organic soap offers several benefits for both your skin and the environment. Here are some key benefits of using organic soap:

1. Gentle on the Skin: Organic soap is made with natural and gentle ingredients, such as plant-based oils, botanical extracts, and essential oils. It lacks harsh chemicals and synthetic additives that can strip the skin of its natural oils and cause irritation or dryness. It is suitable for all skin types, including sensitive and allergy-prone skin.

2. Nourishing and Moisturizing: Organic soap is often formulated with moisturizing oils, such as coconut oil, shea butter, or olive oil, which help to hydrate and nourish the skin. These natural ingredients can leave your skin feeling soft, smooth, and supple.

3. Free from Harsh Chemicals: Organic soap is free from harsh chemicals like sulfates, parabens, phthalates, and artificial fragrances, which can potentially cause skin irritation, allergies, or other adverse effects. Choosing organic soap reduces your exposure to these potentially harmful substances.

4. Environmentally Friendly: Organic soap is typically made with sustainably sourced ingredients and produced using environmentally friendly practices. It often comes in minimal or recyclable packaging, reducing waste and promoting eco-conscious living.

5. Cruelty-Free: Many organic soap brands are cruelty-free, meaning they do not test their products on animals. By using organic soap, you can support ethical and compassionate manufacturing practices.

6. Therapeutic Benefits: Organic soaps often incorporate essential oils and botanical extracts known for their therapeutic properties. These ingredients can provide aromatherapy benefits, such as relaxation, stress relief, or invigoration, depending on the chosen scents.

7. Variety and Customization: Organic soap comes in a wide range of scents, colors, and textures, allowing you to find or create a soap that suits your preferences. You can choose from a variety of natural fragrances derived from essential oils, and even experiment with adding herbs, exfoliants, or other beneficial ingredients to customize your soap.

8. Supporting Local and Artisan Businesses: Choosing organic soap from local or artisan soap makers supports small businesses and contributes to local economies. It encourages the growth of sustainable and community-oriented practices.

By opting for organic soap, you can enjoy the benefits of a gentle, nourishing, and eco-friendly cleansing experience while taking care of your skin and making a positive impact on the environment.

Chapter 3

Essential Ingredients

When making organic soap, the essential ingredients typically include:

1. Base Oils/Fats: These are the main ingredients that provide the soap's cleansing properties and nourishment for the skin. Common base oils used in organic soap making include:

- Olive oil
- Coconut oil
- Palm oil (sustainable source)
- Shea butter
- Cocoa butter
- Avocado oil
- Sweet almond oil
- Castor oil
- Sunflower oil

2. Lye (Sodium Hydroxide): Lye is necessary for the saponification process, which converts the oils into soap. It is important to handle lye with care and follow proper safety guidelines when working with it.

3. Distilled Water: Water is used to dissolve the lye and combine it with the oils/fats during the soap-making process.

4. Essential Oils: Essential oils are derived from plants and add fragrance to the soap. They can also provide therapeutic benefits. Popular essential oils used in organic soap making include lavender, tea tree, peppermint, citrus oils, eucalyptus, and chamomile.

5. Natural Colorants: Natural colorants are derived from plants, minerals, or clays and can be used to give the soap a desired color. Some examples include spirulina powder, cocoa powder, turmeric, activated charcoal, mica powder, and clay.

6. Botanicals and Additives: Additional ingredients can be added to provide various properties and benefits to the soap, such as exfoliation or skin-soothing effects. Some common botanicals and additives used in organic soap making include:

- Herbs (e.g., lavender buds, rose petals, calendula petals)
- Oatmeal
- Honey
- Aloe vera gel/juice
- Yogurt
- Silk fibers
- Kaolin clay
- Bentonite clay
- Coconut milk
- Jojoba beads

It's important to use high-quality, organic, and sustainably sourced ingredients when making organic soap to maintain the integrity of the organic label. The specific combination and quantities of these ingredients can vary depending on the desired properties and recipe of the soap.

Chapter 4

Organic Soap Making Techniques

There are several techniques used for making organic soap, each with its own advantages and requirements. Here are some common techniques used in organic soap making:

1. Cold Process: Cold process soap making involves mixing oils/fats with lye (sodium hydroxide) and allowing the mixture to undergo saponification at room temperature. The soap mixture is then poured into molds and left to cure for several weeks. This technique provides flexibility in formulating recipes and allows for the incorporation of a wide range of ingredients.

2. Hot Process: Hot process soap making involves a similar process to cold process

soap making, but with the addition of heat to speed up the saponification process. The soap mixture is heated and cooked, typically in a slow cooker or double boiler, to accelerate saponification. Hot process soap is ready to use immediately or after a short curing period.

3. Melt and Pour: Melt and pour soap making involves melting pre-made soap bases, which are typically glycerin-based, and adding colorants, fragrances, and other additives. The melted soap mixture is then poured into molds and left to harden. This technique is convenient and doesn't require working with lye, making it suitable for beginners or those who prefer a simpler process.

4. Rebatching: Rebatching, also known as hand-milling, involves grating or chopping pre-made soap and melting it down with additional oils, herbs, or additives. The mixture is then poured into molds and

allowed to harden. This technique is useful for salvaging imperfect or failed batches of soap and allows for creative customization.

5. Transparent Soap: Transparent soap making involves using alcohol, sugar, or other solvents to dissolve soap crystals, resulting in a clear, transparent soap. This technique requires precision and specialized ingredients.

6. Hot Process Liquid Soap: Hot process liquid soap making is similar to hot process soap making but with the aim of creating liquid soap instead of solid bars. This technique involves cooking the soap mixture with water or other liquids until the soap is fully saponified.

Each technique requires specific equipment, safety precautions, and knowledge of ingredient properties and proportions. It's essential to carefully follow instructions, use proper protective gear, and understand the specific requirements of the chosen technique to ensure successful and safe organic soap making.

Chapter 5

Formulating organic Soap Recipes

Formulating organic soap recipes involves selecting the right combination of oils, butters, essential oils, botanicals, and other additives to create a soap that is gentle, nourishing, and suits your preferences. Here are some steps to help you formulate your own organic soap recipe:

1. Understand the Properties of Oils: Familiarize yourself with the properties and characteristics of different oils used in soap making. Each oil has its own fatty acid composition and properties that contribute to the final soap's cleansing, moisturizing, and lathering abilities. Some oils are more suited for specific skin types or desired soap qualities. Common oils used in organic soap making include olive oil, coconut oil, palm oil, shea butter, cocoa butter, and more.

2. Determine the Desired Soap Qualities: Consider the qualities you want your soap to have. Do you want a soap that produces a rich lather? Are you looking for a soap with excellent moisturizing properties? Would you like it to have a creamy or hard texture? Determining the desired qualities will guide your selection of oils and additives.

3. Create a Balanced Recipe: Start by selecting a combination of oils that will provide a good balance of cleansing, moisturizing, and lathering properties. This can involve using a combination of oils with different fatty acid profiles to achieve the desired balance. Use soap calculators or formulation tools available online to calculate the appropriate amounts of oils and lye needed for your recipe while considering factors like the desired superfat percentage (the amount of oils left unsaponified).

4. Consider Additives and Botanicals: Explore the incorporation of additional ingredients to enhance the soap's properties and provide additional benefits. This can include essential oils for fragrance and therapeutic benefits, botanicals like dried herbs, flowers, or clays for exfoliation or color, and other additives such as milk, honey, or oatmeal for added moisturizing or soothing effects.

5. Test and Adjust: Once you have formulated your soap recipe, it's important to conduct small test batches to assess the performance and qualities of the soap. Observe factors like lather, cleansing ability, moisturization, and fragrance. If necessary, make adjustments to the recipe by altering the oil ratios, superfatting percentage, or additives until you achieve the desired results.

6. Document and Track: Keep a record of your soap recipes, including the specific

ingredients, proportions, and any adjustments made. This will help you replicate successful recipes and make further modifications if needed.

Remember to always follow safety guidelines, such as wearing appropriate protective gear and handling lye with caution, during the soap-making process. Experimenting with different oils, additives, and botanicals can lead to unique and personalized organic soap recipes that cater to your specific preferences and skincare needs.

Chapter 6

Scenting and Coloring Naturally

Scenting and coloring organic soap naturally can be achieved using various plant-based ingredients. Here are some methods for scenting and coloring organic soap naturally:

1. Essential Oils: Essential oils derived from plants are a popular choice for natural soap scenting. They not only provide pleasing fragrances but also offer therapeutic benefits. Select essential oils that are skin-safe and suitable for soap making. Some commonly used essential oils for soap scenting include lavender, tea tree, eucalyptus, citrus oils, peppermint, and chamomile. Add the essential oils to your soap mixture during the soap-making process, following recommended usage rates for safe and balanced scenting.

2. Herbs and Botanicals: Dried herbs and botanicals can add subtle scents and natural color to your soap. They can be infused into the oils used for soap making or added directly to the soap mixture. Some popular herbs and botanicals for scenting and coloring include lavender buds, rose petals, chamomile flowers, calendula petals, and dried citrus peels. To infuse the herbs, steep them in warm oils for several hours or overnight before incorporating the infused oils into your soap recipe.

3. Natural Colorants: Various natural ingredients can be used to add color to your organic soap. Here are some examples of natural colorants:

- Plant Powders: Powders derived from plants, such as spirulina, turmeric, beetroot, cocoa powder, or matcha, can be added directly to the soap mixture to achieve different shades of green, yellow, red, brown, or even black.

- Clays: Cosmetic clays, such as French green clay, kaolin clay, or pink clay, not only add color but also provide additional detoxifying or exfoliating properties to the soap. They can be added to the soap mixture or used as a swirl on the top layer.

- Herbal Infusions: Infusing herbs, spices, or teas into oils can produce subtle color variations in the soap. For example, infusing annatto seeds in oil can create a warm yellow color, while infusing hibiscus flowers can result in a pink or reddish hue.

4. Natural Exfoliants: Ingredients like finely ground oatmeal, coffee grounds, poppy seeds, or dried citrus zest can add texture and gentle exfoliation to your soap. These natural exfoliants not only enhance the visual appeal but also offer a mild scrubbing effect when used on the skin.

When incorporating scents and colors into your organic soap, be mindful of the desired concentration and ensure that the ingredients used are skin-safe, natural, and compatible with soap making. It's always recommended to conduct small test batches to determine the desired scent and color intensity before scaling up production.

Chapter 7

Specialty Soaps and Techniques of organic Soap

Organic soap offers a wide range of specialty soaps and techniques that can elevate your soap-making experience. Here are some specialty soaps and techniques you can explore in organic soap making:

1. Specialty Soap Bars:

   - Herbal Soaps: Infusing herbs, flowers, or botanicals into your soap can provide additional benefits and visual appeal. For example, you can create soothing chamomile soap, invigorating rosemary soap, or exfoliating lavender soap.

   - Moisturizing Soaps: Incorporate nourishing ingredients like shea butter, cocoa butter, or avocado oil to create soap bars that offer intense moisturization for dry or sensitive skin.

   - Exfoliating Soaps: Add natural exfoliants such as ground coffee, oatmeal, or poppy seeds to create soaps that gently remove dead skin cells and leave the skin smooth and refreshed.

- Specialty Scented Soaps: Experiment with unique scent combinations using essential oils or natural fragrance oils to create captivating scents like citrus and ginger, vanilla and lavender, or mint and eucalyptus.

2. Swirling and Layering Techniques:

- Swirling: Use different colors of soap batter and create swirl patterns by pouring them into the mold in a controlled manner. You can achieve beautiful designs like the popular "hanger swirl," "in-the-pot swirl," or "Taiwan swirl."

- Layering: Pouring different layers of differently colored soap batter into the mold allows you to create visually stunning layered designs. You can experiment with vertical layers, diagonal layers, or even embed botanicals or exfoliants in between layers.

3. Embeds and Inclusions:

   - Embeds: Embed small soap shapes, such as flowers, hearts, or seashells, into your soap bars. These can be created separately and placed strategically within the soap mold before pouring the main soap batter.

   - Inclusions: Add decorative elements like dried flowers, botanicals, or exfoliants on the top layer of your soap bars. This creates an eye-catching visual effect and enhances the overall appearance of the soap.

4. Liquid Soaps:

   - Castile Soap: Experiment with making liquid soap, particularly Castile soap, which is traditionally made from olive oil. Castile soap can be used for various purposes, such as handwashing, body wash, or even as a gentle household cleaner.

5. Shampoo Bars:

   - Formulate shampoo bars using gentle cleansing ingredients and hair-nourishing oils. Customize the recipe with essential oils that promote healthy hair and scalp, such as rosemary, lavender, or tea tree oil.

Remember to research and follow proper safety guidelines, including working with lye safely, using appropriate protective gear, and properly labeling your specialty soaps. Exploring these specialty soaps and techniques can add creativity and uniqueness to your organic soap-making endeavors:

Chapter 8

Troubleshooting and Common Challenges

Making organic soaps can be a rewarding process, but like any craft, it can come with its own set of challenges. Here are some common troubleshooting and challenges you may encounter when making organic soaps, along with possible solutions:

1. Soap Not Hardening:
   - Possible Causes: Insufficient lye, inaccurate measurements, or using oils with high levels of unsaponifiables.
   - Solutions: Double-check your measurements and ensure accurate lye calculations. Make sure you are using fresh and accurately weighed ingredients. If using oils with high unsaponifiable content, consider adjusting your recipe or using different oils.

2. Soap Cracking:

- Possible Causes: Rapid cooling, excessive moisture loss, or incomplete saponification.

- Solutions: Allow the soap to cool slowly and evenly. Cover it with a towel or blanket to insulate it during the initial cooling phase. Avoid moving or disturbing the soap while it is setting. Check that the soap has completed saponification before unmolding. If necessary, give the soap more time to cure before use.

3. Soap Separation or Ricing:

- Possible Causes: Overheating the oils or lye solution, adding ingredients at improper temperatures, or using incompatible ingredients.

- Solutions: Maintain appropriate temperatures when combining the oils and lye. Slowly add and incorporate ingredients into the soap batter while ensuring they are at a compatible temperature. If ricing occurs, use a stick blender to blend the soap mixture until smooth.

4. Soap Discoloration:

- Possible Causes: Certain oils or additives can cause discoloration over time. Exposure to light, heat, or air can also impact color stability.

- Solutions: Use oils and additives that are less likely to cause discoloration, or embrace the natural color changes as part of the soap's character. Store soaps in a cool, dark place to minimize color fading or changes.

5. Fragrance Fading:

- Possible Causes: Some fragrances, particularly those derived from natural essential oils, can fade over time or be affected by the soap-making process.

- Solutions: Use fragrance oils specifically designed for soap making if you desire long-lasting scents. Experiment with scent blending and try higher concentrations of fragrance oils to achieve a stronger aroma.

6. Mold and Mildew Growth:

- Possible Causes: Insufficient curing time, excess moisture in the soap, or improper storage.

- Solutions: Ensure your soap has ample time to cure and dry before use. Avoid storing soaps in humid or damp conditions. Use a soap dish or tray that allows proper drainage and air circulation to prevent mold and mildew growth.

Remember that troubleshooting soap-making issues often requires experimentation, patience, and attention to detail. Document your process, make small adjustments, and keep track of what works best for your recipes. With practice, you'll become more adept at addressing challenges and creating high-quality organic soaps.

Chapter 9

Packaging and Presentation of organic soap

Packaging and presentation play a significant role in the overall appeal and marketability of your organic soap products. Here are some considerations and ideas for packaging and presenting your organic soaps:

1. Labeling:

   - Include the name of your brand or product, the soap's name or scent, a list of ingredients, and any relevant certifications (e.g., organic, vegan, cruelty-free).

   - Ensure that the label design aligns with your brand's aesthetic and conveys the natural and organic qualities of your soap.

   - Consider using eco-friendly and sustainable labeling materials, such as recycled paper or biodegradable options.

2. Wrapping:

- Wrap individual soap bars in eco-friendly materials like recycled paper, tissue paper, or fabric. This adds a touch of elegance and protects the soap during transportation and handling.

- Use natural twine, hemp cord, or raffia ribbon to secure the wrapping and add a rustic or organic touch.

3. Packaging Materials:

- Choose packaging materials that are eco-friendly, recyclable, or biodegradable to align with the ethos of organic soap making.

- Consider using cardboard boxes, kraft paper sleeves, glassine bags, or reusable tins or containers.

- If using plastic packaging, opt for biodegradable or compostable options made from plant-based materials.

4. Visual Appeal:

- Showcase the unique qualities of your organic soap through thoughtful presentation.

- Consider adding decorative elements like dried flowers, herbs, or botanicals to the packaging for an attractive visual touch.

- Experiment with different textures, colors, and patterns to create a visually appealing and cohesive brand identity.

5. Branding:

- Develop a consistent and recognizable brand identity through your packaging design.

- Use a logo, specific font styles, and color schemes that align with your brand's image and values.

- Create a cohesive packaging design across your soap line to establish brand recognition and a professional look.

6. Informational Inserts:

- Include informational inserts or cards that provide additional details about your organic soap, such as its benefits, usage instructions, or special features.

- Consider including a QR code or website link for customers to access more information or to connect with your brand.

7. Sustainability:

- Highlight the eco-friendly aspects of your packaging, such as recyclability or reusability, to appeal to environmentally conscious consumers.

- Clearly communicate your commitment to sustainability and the use of natural and organic ingredients on your packaging and marketing materials.

Remember to comply with any labeling and packaging regulations specific to your country or region. Additionally, consider conducting market research to identify packaging trends and preferences among your target audience. The goal is to create packaging and presentation that reflects the quality, naturalness, and appeal of your organic soap products while capturing the attention and interest of potential customers.

Chapter 10

Safety and Good Manufacturing

Safety and good manufacturing practices are crucial when producing organic soap to ensure the quality, efficacy, and safety of the final product. Here are some key considerations for maintaining safety and implementing good manufacturing practices for organic soap production:

1. Personal Safety:

   - Wear appropriate protective gear, such as gloves, goggles, and aprons, when handling ingredients like lye or essential oils.

   - Work in a well-ventilated area to minimize exposure to fumes or airborne particles.

   - Follow safety guidelines and instructions provided by manufacturers for handling and storing ingredients.

2. Cleanliness and Sanitation:

- Keep your soap-making area clean and free from contaminants.

- Wash your hands thoroughly before and during the soap-making process to prevent the introduction of bacteria or impurities.

- Disinfect equipment, utensils, and work surfaces regularly to maintain hygiene.

3. Ingredient Quality:

- Source high-quality organic ingredients from reputable suppliers to ensure their purity and authenticity.

- Conduct thorough research on the properties and handling requirements of each ingredient to ensure safe and effective use.

- Be aware of potential allergens and sensitivities associated with certain ingredients, and label your products accordingly.

4. Recipe Development:

- Use reliable and tested recipes from trusted sources, or formulate your own recipes with a solid understanding of the properties and interactions of the ingredients.

   - Conduct small-scale testing before scaling up production to ensure the desired outcome and safety of the soap.

5. Proper Handling of Lye:
   - Handle lye with caution, as it is a caustic substance.
   - Always add lye to liquid (such as water or milk) and never the other way around to minimize the risk of splashing.
   - Follow proper lye safety guidelines, including wearing protective gear and avoiding inhaling fumes.

6. Batch Documentation and Record Keeping:
   - Maintain detailed records of each soap batch, including the ingredients used, their quantities, manufacturing dates, and any special notes or observations.

- Keep track of expiration dates or recommended shelf life for each batch to ensure product freshness and quality.

7. Packaging and Labeling Compliance:
- Adhere to labeling regulations specific to your country or region, including ingredient lists, weight or volume declarations, and safety warnings.
- Clearly communicate any potential allergens or sensitizing ingredients on the label.
- Include proper storage instructions and precautions for consumers.

8. Good Manufacturing Practices (GMP):
- Implement GMP guidelines, which encompass a range of practices aimed at maintaining product quality, cleanliness, and safety throughout the manufacturing process.
- Establish standard operating procedures (SOPs) for various aspects of soap production, including ingredient handling,

equipment cleaning, and quality control measures.

   - Regularly review and update your SOPs to reflect best practices and ensure consistency in production.

It's important to stay updated on current regulations, guidelines, and best practices related to organic soap production in your specific location. Consulting with regulatory authorities or industry experts can provide valuable insights and help ensure compliance with safety standards.

Chapter 11

Exploring Soap Variations

Exploring soap variations in organic soap making allows you to create a diverse range of products with different qualities and benefits. Here are some soap variations you can explore in your organic soap-making journey:

1. Herbal Infused Soaps:

   - Incorporate dried herbs, flowers, or botanicals into your soap recipes to add fragrance, texture, and potential therapeutic properties. Examples include lavender-infused soap, chamomile-infused soap, or calendula-infused soap.

2. Exfoliating Soaps:

   - Add natural exfoliants like ground coffee, oatmeal, sea salt, or crushed fruit seeds to create soaps that gently slough away dead skin cells, leaving the skin smooth and refreshed.

3. Moisturizing Soaps:

   - Include nourishing ingredients such as shea butter, cocoa butter, mango butter, avocado oil, or jojoba oil to create soaps that provide intense moisturization and hydration for dry or sensitive skin.

4. Aromatherapy Soaps:

   - Utilize essential oils with various therapeutic properties to create soaps that promote relaxation, rejuvenation, or upliftment. Examples include lavender and chamomile for relaxation, citrus oils for energizing, or eucalyptus for a refreshing experience.

5. Milk-based Soaps:

   - Use milk, such as goat's milk or plant-based milk alternatives, as a base for your soap. Milk adds creaminess, moisturizing properties, and can provide a luxurious lather.

6. Specialty Oil Soaps:

   - Experiment with different specialty oils known for their unique properties. For instance, castor oil can create a rich lather, while coconut oil adds cleansing and bubbly qualities. Olive oil is known for its moisturizing properties.

7. Shampoo Bars:

   - Formulate soap bars specifically designed for hair washing. Use hair-nourishing oils like argan oil or jojoba oil, and incorporate beneficial ingredients like herbal extracts or essential oils known to support healthy hair and scalp.

8. Decorative and Artistic Soaps:

   - Explore creative techniques like swirling, layering, or embedding to create visually appealing and artistic soap designs. These soaps can be eye-catching and make great gifts or decorative bathroom pieces.

9. Specialty Soaps for Skin Conditions:

- Develop soaps tailored to specific skin conditions, such as acne-prone skin, sensitive skin, or eczema. Choose ingredients and essential oils known for their soothing, healing, or balancing properties.

Remember to document your recipes and variations, noting the quantities of ingredients used and any observations regarding scent, texture, or performance. This way, you can replicate successful variations and refine your recipes over time. Have fun exploring these soap variations and discovering unique combinations that suit your preferences and the needs of your customers.

Chapter 12

Selling Homemade organic Soap

Selling homemade organic soap can be a rewarding venture. Here are some steps to help you get started:

1. Develop a Unique Selling Proposition:

   - Identify what sets your homemade organic soap apart from others in the market. Determine your target audience and their specific needs or preferences. Highlight the unique qualities, such as organic ingredients, special formulations, or specific benefits of your soap.

2. Ensure Compliance with Regulations:

   - Research and comply with local regulations regarding the sale of cosmetics and handmade soaps. This may include labeling requirements, ingredient disclosures, and safety regulations.

3. Create a Brand and Packaging:
   - Develop a cohesive brand identity that aligns with your values and appeals to your target audience. Choose a memorable brand name, design a logo, and create visually appealing packaging that reflects the natural and organic nature of your soap.

4. Establish a Reliable Supply Chain:
   - Source high-quality organic ingredients from trusted suppliers to ensure consistency and quality in your soap production. Maintain good relationships with suppliers and ensure a steady supply of ingredients.

5. Pricing Your Products:
   - Determine the appropriate pricing for your handmade organic soaps by considering the cost of ingredients, packaging, overhead expenses, and desired profit margins. Research the market to understand pricing trends and competitive pricing for similar products.

6. Build an Online Presence:

- Set up a professional website or an online store where customers can browse and purchase your organic soaps. Showcase your product range, provide detailed product descriptions, and include high-quality product images.

- Leverage social media platforms to create a strong online presence. Share visually appealing content, engage with your audience, and promote your products. Consider using platforms like Instagram, Facebook, or Pinterest, which are popular for visual-based products.

7. Explore Local Sales Channels:

- Attend local craft fairs, farmers markets, or community events to showcase and sell your organic soaps directly to customers. Connect with local retailers or boutiques that align with your brand ethos to explore wholesale opportunities.

8. Leverage Online Marketplaces:

- Consider selling your homemade organic soaps on popular online marketplaces like Etsy, Amazon Handmade, or eBay. These platforms provide access to a large customer base and offer built-in e-commerce functionalities.

9. Focus on Marketing and Promotion:

- Implement effective marketing strategies to create awareness and generate interest in your organic soap products. Utilize online advertising, content marketing, social media influencers, and collaborations with complementary brands or influencers.

- Offer promotions, discounts, or loyalty programs to incentivize repeat purchases and customer loyalty.

10. Provide Excellent Customer Service:

- Deliver exceptional customer service by promptly responding to inquiries, addressing customer concerns or issues, and providing a positive buying experience.

Encourage customer reviews and testimonials to build trust and credibility.

Remember to stay consistent in your product quality, branding, and customer service. Continuously seek feedback from customers and adapt your offerings based on market trends and customer preferences. By focusing on quality, differentiation, and effective marketing strategies, you can successfully sell your homemade organic soaps and build a loyal customer base.